INTERMITTENT FASTING TRANSFORMATION FOR WOMEN:

A Practical Guide to Lose Stubborn Weight, Improve Hormonal Health and Slow Aging

Vivian Blake

Table of contents

Introduction

Chapter One: What is Intermittent Fasting?

Chapter 2: Understanding Hormonal Health

Chapter 3: Getting Started with Intermittent Fasting

Chapter 4 Maintaining Your Intermittent Fasting Transformation

Introduction

We are determined to ignore the most obvious approach, which is to refrain from eating for some time, in a world that looks so anxious for solutions regarding how to lose fat. Intermittent fasting is a very effective method for shedding pounds. According to my professional experience as a dietitian and my personal experience trying out weight loss tactics, I advise clients to use it. Along with saving you a ton of time and money, it is also incredibly beneficial to your health. Better yet, if you can exercise. It almost seems redundant to write an entire book about fasting for weight loss because it makes so much sense. And yet, you've undoubtedly heard the following sayings before:

- The most significant meal of the day is breakfast."

- Your metabolism will slow down if you skip a meal, which will lead to weight gain.

- You'll be so hungry at the next meal that you'll overeat if you don't eat every couple of hours. Before working out, you must fuel your body (with carbohydrates) or you won't have the energy to do so.

- Your blood sugar will drop if you don't eat every few hours, which will cause you to feel weak and faint.

Because we have so little experience with it, the majority of us truly think that when we fast, horrible things will happen to our bodies. However, none of the side effects that individuals worry about before giving fasting a try—weakness, fatigue, mental fog, etc.—occur when you fast. Additionally, it doesn't slow your metabolism; in fact, it has the exact opposite effect, for a variety of reasons that we'll go into great length about in the chapters to come. Worldwide, millions of individuals regularly fast as a part of their religious or cultural rituals, reaping the advantages of better physical and mental health.

But fasting is practically unheard of in our culture. The body requires small, frequent meals throughout the day, according to nutritional professionals as well as every health and fitness publication out there. Meals must never be skipped, and snacks are encouraged. Because of this, we have persuaded ourselves that we need to eat constantly to maintain a healthy weight. Do you truly think that's appropriate? I think the concept is ridiculous and has harmed a lot of individuals. If you weren't doubting it, you probably wouldn't be prepared to try intermittent fasting.

In this book, I want to show you that fasting intermittently is a very safe and efficient approach to reducing weight, and more precisely, shedding body fat while maintaining muscle mass. I want to dispel any worries you might have about skipping meals being detrimental to your health or making you gain weight instead of reducing it. I'll provide you with tips to make your fast successful as well as guidance on how to incorporate intermittent fasting into your daily life. Before you finish this book, I want you to be so convinced of the advantages of fasting and how simple it is to practice it that you decide to try your first 24-hour fast.

Chapter One: What is Intermittent Fasting?

Alternating between eating and fasting times is known as intermittent fasting. If food is ingested at all during the fasting period, it is usually in extremely small amounts. A typical meal is consumed throughout the dining period. Weight loss, better hormonal health, and delayed aging are just a few of the health advantages of this eating pattern that have been demonstrated.

The ability to produce a calorie deficit, which is necessary for weight loss to take place, is one of the key advantages of intermittent fasting for weight loss. Your body uses fat and glucose (sugar) that have been stored for energy when you fast, which causes you to lose weight. Furthermore, intermittent fasting has been demonstrated to enhance insulin sensitivity, which can result in improved blood

Through the promotion of cellular repair and the reduction of inflammation, intermittent fasting can help reduce the aging process. Human growth hormone, which can aid in gaining muscle and lowering body fat, has been demonstrated in studies to be produced more frequently when people practice intermittent fasting. It may also aid in enhancing cognitive function and lowering the risk of chronic illnesses.

Additionally advantageous for hormonal health is intermittent fasting. It can enhance insulin sensitivity and balance hormones, making it simpler for people to lose weight and enhance their general health. Though there are several forms of intermittent fasting, it's crucial to remember that you should always speak with a healthcare provider before beginning a new diet or exercise program.

The eight distinct intermittent fasting strategies

The key difference between intermittent fasting techniques is the length of the fast. We outline the most common techniques.

1. The 12-hour or overnight fast

The most basic kind of fasting is 12 hours. You fast every day for 12 hours, which includes your evening fast. So all you need to do is abstain from eating for a short while before night and after waking up. Breakfast, lunch, and supper are the usual three meals you eat. This seems less like fasting and more like a regular eating plan. The distinction is that you don't snack, which would cut your fasting duration in half. Say you finish eating dinner at 7 o'clock, at which point your fast will begin. After dinner, you could continue munching, which would cut your fasting time in half.

You could believe that this minor difference has no real impact, but you'd be incorrect. In a study of diabetic patients, it was discovered that eating three meals a day and avoiding snacks greatly reduced their weight and brought down their blood sugar levels. The insulin dosage may be decreased concurrently.

What makes this possible?

Your blood sugar and insulin levels increase every time you eat, and it takes some time for them to return to normal. When you often eat, your blood sugar and insulin hardly have time to stabilize in between meals.

Blood sugar and insulin levels only increase three times with only three meals, and they remain within the normal range for the majority of the day. Because of this, eating three meals a day and avoiding snacks already reduces insulin levels and improves insulin resistance (the underlying cause of type 2 diabetes). Keeping insulin levels low also aids in weight loss since insulin not only lowers blood sugar but also acts as a hormone that stores fat. Therefore, even if you do not currently have diabetes, frequent snacking raises your risk; therefore, refraining from it lowers your risk and enhances general health.

Another method of observing a 12-hour fast is to consume only two meals per day—breakfast and dinner. You have two lengthy fasting periods every day in this manner. Many people who prefer to eat breakfast in the morning and want to spend time socializing with family or friends at supper but don't have much time for lunch at work would find this schedule to be convenient.

Advisable for:
- Freshers
- People who want to experience the health benefits of intermittent fasting but don't need to shed a lot of weight

Main advantages
- Breakfast, lunch, and dinner are typically eaten at regular times.
- Reduces the incidence of chronic diseases like diabetes and improves general health

2. The 14/10 fasting

This is another approach that is simple enough for beginners to use right away without any prior fasting expertise is the 14/10 intermittent fast. After a 14-hour fast, you have ten hours to eat. Due to its simplicity and similar health benefits to the well-known 16/8 approach, the 14/10 method is preferred by women who have trouble with lengthier fasting periods. During your eating window, you are permitted to consume two or three meals. You need to space out your meals if you eat three meals a day. You have quite a long interval in between meals when you eat two.

Advisable for:
- Freshers
- Women who have trouble maintaining lengthier fasts

Main advantages
- Easily attainable

- Helps with weight loss

3. The 16/8 Fasting

The most common type of intermittent fasting is 16/8 fasting. Though slightly more complex than the first two, it is still quite user-friendly for beginners. Every day, you eat within an eight-hour window and fast for 16 hours. During this time, most people often consume two meals: either lunch and dinner or breakfast and lunch. You can also eat three meals; you simply need to space them out so that they don't overlap by more than eight hours.

The majority of people may quickly get used to 16/8 and lose weight without feeling hungry. The wonderful thing about this form is that, although being quite easy to complete, you can still anticipate getting results.

According to studies, the 16/8 diet can help people keep their muscle mass while helping them lose weight, increase their insulin sensitivity, and reduce inflammation.

Autophagy should begin after 16 hours of fasting. Numerous health advantages of intermittent fasting result from autophagy, an important recycling process. Although longer fasting periods are more effective at promoting autophagy, this process can already begin after 16 to 18 hours.

The method's possible drawback is that you might not get results as rapidly as someone who follows a more stringent fasting regimen, such as alternate-day fasting. Additionally, you are probably not taking full advantage of fasting's ability to extend your life and fight to age. But if you're new to fasting or prefer eating out frequently with friends and family, this is a perfect form for you!

You can transition to 18/6 intermittent fasting if you've become used to 16/8 fasting and feel that you could fast for extended periods with ease. It simply implies that your fasting period will be two hours longer than it would be if you were fasting according to the 16/8 rule.

Advisable for
- Novices and those who have fasted before
- Individuals who are either normal or somewhat overweight

Main advantages
- Helps with weight loss
- An effective way to lower insulin resistance
- Increases autophagy

4. Warrior diet or OMAD

One-Meal-A-Day is abbreviated as OMAD. As implied by the name, you only eat once every day. Due to its convenience for busy people, most people just eat dinner. You manage to fast for almost 23 hours each day in this way. Ori Hofmekler, a fitness expert, popularized the warrior diet, which is a variation of the OMAD. It involves eating a single large meal in the evening in addition to small amounts of fruits, nuts, and vegetables throughout the day.

The OMAD method of intermittent fasting is highly sophisticated. Even yet, some people find it rather simple, especially if they are not particularly hungry in the morning or at lunch. Choose a time each day when you wish to eat, and fulfill all of your caloric demands at that time, if you want to effectively complete OMAD. And certainly, this meal should have a lot of calories. Depending on your age, sex, height, and level of physical activity, you should consume between 1500 and 2000 calories daily if you decide to follow the OMAD diet.

You should keep in mind that eating too few calories over the long run has been proven to be bad for your health. It could be challenging to eat so much at first, which is normal, but after a few weeks, your body ought to adjust, and it ought to get much simpler to eat a calorie-dense meal. If you still find it difficult to consume this much, this diet might not be the ideal choice for you.

When you just eat once a day, your insulin levels are typically low for the majority of the day. Because of this, OMAD is an effective weight-loss strategy. Additionally, the body enters a state of ketosis as a result of the prolonged fast. Ketone bodies, a byproduct of the metabolic process known as ketosis, serve as an additional fuel source. Because it gives access to fat storage, ketosis is incredibly effective for weight loss. Going the entire day without eating may be quite challenging for some people, which is a drawback to this technique. If you give it a shot and find that you're truly suffering, consider easing into it by gradually extending your fast until you can go most of the day without eating. Practice makes perfect.

Advisable for
- Those familiar with intermittent fasting
- People with busy schedules who can't eat during the day

Main advantages

- Promotes autophagy
- Enables ketosis
- Aids with weight loss

5. The Eat Stop Eat

Similar to OMAD, the Eat Stop Eat approach involves fasting for 24 hours between one meal and the same meal the next day. say, from lunch on one day till lunch on the following day. The key distinction from OMAD is that you only do it once or twice per week as opposed to daily.

Because you only fast once or twice a week, one drawback of this diet is that you can just forget and wake up on your fasting day and start eating. Until it becomes a rigid habit of yours, try placing a reminder on your phone or a post-it note to remind you on your designated fasting day. Committing to the same day(s) every week, such as Sunday and Thursday, will assist establish the habit.

Another drawback is that, in comparison to alternate-day fasting or OMAD, it can take a little longer for you to see any improvements because this isn't happening every day. But don't let that get you down! Any advancement you make on your trip is a huge success.

Advisable for
- People familiar with intermittent fasting
- Those who don't wish to observe daily fasting

Main advantages
- Enables ketosis
- Encourages autophagy

6. The Alternate-Day-Fasting (ADF)

ADF stands for alternate-day fasting. As the name implies, you eat every other day. With ADF, you achieve a fasting time of around 36 hours: From dinner on one day until breakfast on the day after the next. ADF, or alternate-day fasting, is a practice. You eat as the name suggests every other day. Through the use of ADF, you can fast for around 36 hours, from dinner one day to breakfast the following.

Due to the lengthy fasting time, alternate-day fasting is arguably one of the most successful types of intermittent fasting. Numerous studies have demonstrated the effectiveness of this approach in assisting people with weight loss, blood sugar control, blood pressure reduction, and other goals.

Alternate-day fasting is also particularly successful at boosting autophagy, reducing aging symptoms, and even extending longevity, according to studies… According to certain animal studies, lifespan can rise by up to 80%. Alternate-day fasting may seem like a simple practice to begin, but going without food for an entire day might be much more difficult than it seems. When first attempting this strategy, some people, particularly those who now eat for more than 15 hours per day, may truly struggle.

ADF is not for everyone, and you don't need to fast for a long time to get the rewards of IF. Please speak with your doctor first if you decide to try it.

Alternate day fasting with modifications

The only difference between modified alternate-day fasting and alternate-day fasting is that participants have a meal of about 500 calories on their fasting days. However, you shouldn't anticipate experiencing all of the advantages of actual alternate-day fasting even though you will undoubtedly observe improvements using this method. But for those who wish to try alternate-day fasting but find it difficult to make it through the entire day, this modified approach can be a perfect option. Try practicing this form for a while before attempting to advance to a full day's fast.

Advisable for
- People with extensive experience fasting
- People that need to drop a lot of weight
- Those that desire to reverse their diabetes (only after consultation with their GP)

Main advantages
- An incredibly effective way to shed a lot of weight quickly
- Increases autophagy

- Allows for profound ketosis
- Improves insulin sensitivity

7. The 5:2 fasting

Similar to ADF, 5:2 fasting involves only two (non-consecutive) days of fasting per week, with the other five days being spent eating normally. On the days you are fasting, you normally consume 500–600 kcal, though you are also allowed to go without eating entirely. 5:2 is a more sophisticated kind of intermittent fasting, similar to ADF. If you want to try it, please speak with your doctor first.

Advisable for
- People who have fasted before
- Those who don't wish to observe daily fasting

Main advantages
- Improves insulin sensitivity
- Increases autophagy
- Allows for ketosis
- Helps with weight loss

8. Intuitive intermittent fasting or spontaneous meal skipping

Despite not wanting to follow a strict meal plan, many people enjoy intermittent fasting. That's ok! The most crucial aspect is to have regular meal breaks, not necessarily at the same time every day. People who have practiced intermittent fasting for a while and become accustomed to this manner of eating tend to approach it more intuitively.

To eat only when you are truly hungry and to keep eating until you are satisfied is the premise of intuitive intermittent fasting. When it's time to eat but you're not hungry, you decide to forgo the meal. The intuitive version assists you in discovering the intermittent fasting technique that works best for you after you begin experimenting with it. Find out what times of the day fasting is easiest and see how long you can go without eating without getting grumpy.

In conclusion, For women, intermittent fasting can be done in a variety of ways. The initial problem is figuring out which approach works best for you. You may conclude that intermittent fasting is not for you if you force yourself to adhere to a fasting schedule that is not healthy for you. On the other hand, if you discover a strategy that perfectly fits your requirements and timetable, it will quickly become second nature and you won't need to keep an eye on the time.

Establishing reasonable weight loss objectives while taking overall health into account

Any weight reduction journey, including switching to intermittent fasting, should include setting realistic weight loss goals. A realistic objective must be time-bound, meaningful, specific, quantifiable, and feasible (SMART). For instance, "I want to lose 10 pounds in three months by exercising three times a week and using the 16/8 method of intermittent fasting." It's crucial to realize that losing weight is only one component of comprehensive wellness. Even though losing weight can be inspiring, it's not the only crucial component.

In addition to helping people lose weight, intermittent fasting has been demonstrated to increase insulin sensitivity and hormonal balance, and decrease the aging process. Focusing on total health rather than simply weight loss is crucial. It is advised to maintain a balanced lifestyle by paying attention to your eating, exercising, and sleeping patterns. Additionally, it's critical to maintain a good outlook and be nice to yourself, understanding that improving one's weight and general health is a journey and that progress rather than perfection should be the objective.

The objective of losing weight may not be the same for everyone, so it's vital to pay attention to your body. If your body is content with your current weight, it's necessary to concentrate on improving your general health rather than your weight.

Importance of seeking medical advice before beginning any new diet or fitness program.

Before beginning an intermittent fasting transformation or any other new diet or fitness program, it's crucial to speak with a healthcare expert. This is particularly valid if you currently use any medications or have any pre-existing medical issues.

- A healthcare practitioner can assist you in determining whether intermittent fasting is safe for you as well as in creating a strategy that is specific to your requirements and objectives. Additionally, they can offer advice on how to integrate intermittent fasting into your existing diet and exercise plan and track your progress.

- A healthcare practitioner can also assist you in determining any underlying health conditions that might be causing weight gain or making it difficult for you to lose weight. Additionally, they can offer advice on how to deal with any dietary deficits that may result from intermittent fasting.

- A healthcare provider should be consulted to make sure intermittent fasting is safe for you and that it will help you lose weight, enhance your hormonal health, and slow the aging process. They may offer advice on how to include it into your routine, how to keep track of your progress, and how to get the most out of this practice.

Chapter 2: Understanding Hormonal Health

The significance of comprehending hormonal health concerning weight loss and general well-being will be covered in this chapter. We will investigate how hormonal abnormalities can impact weight loss and how IF can assist to restore hormonal balance. The regulation of our metabolism, energy balance and hunger is greatly influenced by hormones. They cooperate to regulate how much energy we consume, how much energy we expend, and how much energy is stored in our bodies.

The pancreas secretes the hormone insulin, which aids in controlling blood sugar levels. When we eat, it is released and aids in the transportation of glucose into our cells for energy. Our cells may become insulin-resistant when we consume too much or too frequently, which can result in excessive blood sugar levels and weight gain.

- A hormone generated by the stomach called ghrelin alerts the brain to hunger. Before meals, ghrelin levels rise, and thereafter, they decline. We feel hungry and are more inclined to eat more than we need when ghrelin levels are high, which can result in weight gain.

- The hormone leptin, which is made by fat cells, tells the brain to suppress the appetite and increase energy expenditure. Leptin production declines as we lose weight, making it more difficult to keep weight off.

- The adrenal glands produce the hormone cortisol, which plays a role in the body's reaction to stress. Increased hunger and weight gain are two effects of high cortisol levels.

By balancing these hormones, intermittent fasting can aid in weight reduction by promoting weight loss, but it's also important to understand how these hormones can also lead to weight gain.

 Unbalanced hormones might also make it harder to lose weight. For instance, a person may find it more difficult to lose weight even with diet and exercise if they have a thyroid condition that impairs the thyroid gland's capacity to generate hormones that control metabolism.

Overall, hormones regulate weight in a complicated and linked manner, and hormonal abnormalities can make it challenging to both lose weight and keep it off and maintain a healthy weight. The hormonal balance can be improved and weight loss can be aided by intermittent fasting.

The connection between hormonal imbalance and weight gain

Weight gain, however, is a distinct and obvious symptom that you can see when you look in the mirror. Hormones can cause all sorts of damage to your body without you realizing it. The following are some possible causes of your current hormone imbalance.

1. Menopause

Menopause often begins in women between the ages of 45 and 55. When this happens, a woman stops menstruation as a result of the estrogen hormone's reduction. At this time, a drop in estrogen can also result in weight gain. Your thighs and hips are the typical places where these additional pounds end up. Men's testosterone levels decline as they become older, which causes their body fat and muscle mass to grow. Weight growth is particularly concerning because carrying too much weight around your middle can cause Type 2 diabetes, heart disease, and breathing issues. Additionally, carrying extra weight can make you more susceptible to some cancers.

2. Hypothyroidism

You have hypothyroidism if your body doesn't create enough thyroid hormones. The thyroid is a little gland at the base of your neck that regulates hormones crucial to your well-being. It guarantees that each of your organs has sufficient energy to perform. You may gain weight if your thyroid isn't producing enough of the energy your body needs to function.

3. Endometriosis

Endometrial tissue, which is normally present on the inside of the uterus, can develop outside of the uterine lining as a result of the disorder endometriosis. The ovaries or fallopian tubes may also become infected by this tissue. Extreme discomfort is experienced, especially during menstruation. Although pelvic pain is the most typical symptom of endometriosis, bloating, and weight gain are also frequent. Endometriosis is classified as an "estrogen-dependent disease," which means that progesterone levels are too low and estrogen levels are too high. Weight increase may be correlated with estrogen dominance.

4. PCOS

The polycystic ovarian syndrome is a hormonal abnormality that is comparable to endometriosis (PCOS). Due to the similarities in their symptoms, including bloating, weight gain, and painful periods, they are frequently confused for one another. Although it is unclear whether PCOS always results in initial weight gain, your symptoms may be more severe and challenging to treat if you are heavier. In this instance, persons with PCOS have hormonal imbalances such as high levels of androgen and insulin resistance, which increases the risk of type II diabetes.

Hormonal effects of intermittent fasting

It has been demonstrated that intermittent fasting has advantageous impacts on hormones that support weight loss and enhance general health.

- Improving insulin sensitivity is one of the key advantages of intermittent fasting, which can result in better blood sugar regulation and weight loss. Intermittent fasting can lower insulin levels and improve insulin sensitivity, which may assist to lessen the risk of type 2 diabetes, according to studies.

- Ghrelin levels can be decreased by intermittent fasting, which can result in a decrease in appetite and weight loss. Ghrelin, the hormone that alerts the brain to hunger, has been shown in studies to be reduced by intermittent fasting.

- Additionally, intermittent fasting can improve leptin sensitivity, which can boost calorie expenditure and promote weight loss. According to studies, intermittent fasting might enhance the body's level of leptin, which makes it simpler to maintain a healthy weight.

- Lowering cortisol levels with intermittent fasting may also aid in weight loss and improve general health. Intermittent fasting has been shown in studies to lower cortisol levels, which is good for both weight loss and general health.

It is significant to note that depending on the person and the type of intermittent fasting strategy utilized, the effects of intermittent fasting on hormones can change. Before beginning intermittent fasting, talk to a medical expert, and have them check your hormone levels periodically to make sure it's safe and effective for you.

Chapter 3: Getting Started with Intermittent Fasting

This chapter will offer a step-by-step tutorial for beginning intermittent fasting, including details on selecting the best approach, creating a schedule, organizing meals, and overcoming hunger and cravings.

Choosing the most effective technique of intermittent fasting for you

You probably have a lot of experience with intermittent fasting. If you've ever had dinner, slept in late, and then skipped meals until lunch the next day, you've likely fasted for at least 16 hours. Some people eat in this manner out of instinct. Simply put, they are not hungry in the morning. You might wish to start with the 16/8 approach because it is widely regarded as the easiest and most enduring form of intermittent fasting. If the fast goes well and you feel good, you might want to proceed to more difficult fasts like consuming only 500–600 calories once or twice a week or going without food for 24 hours (5:2 diet).

Another strategy is to just abstain from eating whenever it's convenient, skipping meals occasionally when you're not hungry or don't have time to prepare food. You can reap at least some of the benefits of intermittent fasting without adhering to a planned diet. Try out various strategies until you find one that suits your needs and interests.

Establishing and adhering to a schedule

The significance of creating and adhering to a schedule when beginning intermittent fasting will be covered in this section.

1. Picking a schedule that suits your needs

It's crucial to pick a schedule that works with your daily schedule and way of life. The 16/8 approach, for instance, might be a better fit for you than the Warrior Diet if you enjoy eating breakfast.

2. Getting used to fasting gradually

It's crucial to progressively introduce fasting into your life. If you've never fasted before, for instance, you can begin with 12 hours and work your way up to 16 hours.

3. Maintaining the schedule

It's crucial to maintain the schedule as much as you can after choosing one and acclimating to it gradually. Although first difficult, doing this consistently over time will make it easier.

4. Being adaptable

It's crucial to keep in mind that life occasionally interferes with our plans, so you might need to adjust them. To avoid turning one hiccup into a pattern of not keeping to the timetable, it's crucial to get back on track as quickly as you can.

5. Progress tracking

Keeping tabs on your development might help you stay inspired and on course. This can involve keeping note of your weight, body measurements, and emotional state. The effectiveness of intermittent fasting depends on creating and adhering to a plan, but it's also critical to be adaptable and keep in mind that the goal is progress rather than perfection.

6. Planning and preparing meals

The significance of meal preparation and planning when adhering to an intermittent fasting schedule will be covered in this section.

- Making a food plan: Making a meal plan ahead of time will ensure that you consume wholesome, filling meals throughout your eating window. This can involve making plans for breakfast, lunch, dinner, and, if necessary, snacks.

- Getting meals ready in advance: Meals that are prepared ahead of time might save time and help you stay on schedule. This can be done by cooking and portioning out meals for the following day or by organizing the meals for the upcoming week on the weekends.

- Having wholesome snacks available: Having healthy snacks on hand throughout your fasting time will help you control urges and prevent overeating. Nuts, seeds, and raw veggies are a few examples of healthful snacks.

- Maintaining hydration: Water, tea, and other non-caloric beverages can all assist to quell your appetite while you're fasting. Hydration is also crucial.

- Test-driving various foods: The chance to try out various foods and see which ones are best for you can be found in intermittent fasting. For example, you might experiment with brand-new ingredients, techniques, and recipes.

It's vital to remember that meal preparation and planning are crucial for the success of intermittent fasting. By organizing and preparing your meals ahead of time, you can make sure you acquire the nutrients you require throughout your eating window.

Dealing with hunger and cravings during intermittent fasting

1. Managing hunger and cravings

Dealing with hunger and cravings can be one of the intermittent fasting's major obstacles. Keeping hydrated, stocking up on nutritious snacks, and engaging in mindfulness exercises like deep breathing or meditation are some ways to control hunger and cravings.

2. Finding alternatives

It can be easier to feel full without breaking your fast if you can find alternatives to your favorite high-calorie items. For instance, instead of reaching for a candy bar if you have a sweet tooth, try a piece of fruit or a tiny amount of dark chocolate.

3. Keeping trigger foods at bay

Knowing which foods trigger binges or overeating will help you stick to your intermittent fasting regimen.

4. Being aware of the distinction between hunger and cravings

It's important to distinguish between cravings and hunger, which are two different physical experiences. Cravings are frequently driven by emotions or habits.

5. Self-distraction

It can be useful to learn techniques for diverting your attention from cravings and hunger.

6. Gradual modification

Reduced hunger and cravings can also be achieved by gradually adjusting to the fasting schedule. Starting with shorter fasts, you can gradually lengthen them as time goes on.

7. Consuming nutrient-rich food:

Nutrient-dense foods can help you feel full and satisfied for a longer period when consumed during your eating window.

8. Consistency

Your body will become accustomed to the pattern and experience fewer hunger pangs and cravings as a result of your continued consistency with your intermittent fasting regimen.

9. Being adaptable

Your fasting schedule should be flexible. It's permissible to break your fast early or take a small snack if you're feeling very peckish. The most crucial step is to pay attention to your body and make any necessary adjustments.

Incorporating exercise into intermittent fasting

Including exercise in your intermittent fasting regimen might help you lose weight and get healthier overall. But it's crucial to approach exercise sustainably and safely. The following advice will help you add exercise to your intermittent fasting schedule:

1. Timing

To reduce feelings of exhaustion and hunger, time your workout around your meal window. As your body has more energy and nutrients available to fuel your workout, you may also find it advantageous to exercise after breaking your fast.

2. Exercise Type

For weight loss and overall health, combining cardio and strength exercise is beneficial.

3. Observe your body

Pay attention to how your body feels while exercising and after. It may be beneficial to take a break or lower the intensity of your workout if you are feeling very weak or exhausted.

4. Gradual increment

You can reduce your risk of injury and exhaustion by gradually increasing the length and intensity of your workouts.

5. Speak with a specialist:

To develop a safe and efficient fitness routine that is customized to your unique requirements and goals, speak with a healthcare expert or a personal trainer.

6. Remain hydrated

To stay hydrated and maintain your body's function throughout exercise, it's crucial to drink enough water before, during, and after physical activity.

7. Get enough sleep:

Sleep is essential for general health and can enhance athletic performance. Sleep for 7-9 hours every night.

Tracking progress and making changes

It's crucial to keep track of your success and tweak your intermittent fasting schedule to achieve your weight loss and health objectives. Here are some pointers for keeping track of results and making changes.:

1. Monitor your development

Log your meals and snacks in a journal or keep a food diary. You'll be able to monitor your intake and spot any places where you might need to make changes as a result.

2. Maintain a weight log

Weigh yourself frequently and keep track of any weight changes. It's vital to keep in mind that weight loss may not occur linearly and to concentrate on long-term success rather than short-term swings.

3. Body composition evaluation

Since muscle weighs more than fat, measuring your body composition might help you get a more accurate picture of your progress.

4. Pay attention to your energy levels:

Throughout the day, keep an eye on your energy level and note any changes. Making changes to your fasting schedule or food plan may be worthwhile if you experience prolonged fatigue or sluggishness.

5. Observe your body

Pay attention to the cues coming from your body and modify them as necessary. It can be worthwhile considering changes to your routine if you are extremely hungry or are having problems keeping to your fasting schedule.

6. Speak with a specialist:

To make sure your intermittent fasting regimen is secure and suitable for you, speak with a medical expert or a qualified dietitian.

You can make your intermittent fasting regimen safe and successful for you while also achieving your weight reduction and health goals by keeping track of your progress and adjusting as necessary.

Chapter 4 Maintaining Your Intermittent Fasting Transformation

1. Follow your planned fasting schedule

Make sure you adhere to the fasting and eating windows that you have established for yourself because consistency is important in IF. This will facilitate the routine formation and make it simpler for you to stick to your goal.

2. Prepare a nutritious menu

To support your general health and weight loss objectives, it's crucial to consume balanced, nutrient-rich meals within your eating windows. Be sure to emphasize entire foods, such as fruits and vegetables, lean meats, and healthy fats. Steer clear of processed foods, sugary beverages, and excessive alcohol consumption.

3. Remain hydrated

During fasting periods, drinking plenty of water, herbal tea, and other low-calorie liquids will keep you hydrated and may help you feel less hungry. Aim for 8 glasses of water a day minimum, and up to more if you're exercising.

4. Do not snack

Snacking while fasting can undermine your IF objectives and keep you from experiencing the benefits of the strategy. If you're feeling peckish, try sipping on some water, a low-calorie beverage, or doing something pleasant to divert your attention from eating.

5. Add in physical activity

You can boost your general health, maintain weight loss, and increase your metabolism with regular exercise. Select exercises like weightlifting, yoga, or walking that you can maintain over the long term.

6. Keep from overeating

It's crucial to avoid overeating during your eating windows because doing so can negate the advantages of IF. Pay attention to your hunger and fullness cues when you eat and do it slowly and carefully.

Printed in Great Britain
by Amazon